This Book Belongs To:

_____

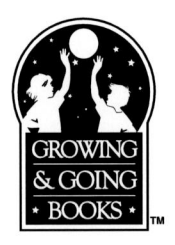

www.healthylivingforkids.com

Fit Kids, Strong Kids

Safe Kids, Smart Kids

Hungry Kids, Healthy Kids

Clean Kids, Happy Kids

Copyright ©2005 Frederic Thomas Inc., Naples, Florida.
"Growing & Going Books" is a Trademark of Frederic Thomas Inc.

Image Credits – Image Credits – Eye Ubiquitous/CORBIS: ©Bennett Dean p13tr; Getty Images: p15tl, Colin Hawkins p23tl; Photo Researchers, Inc.: ©Scimat p7cl, ©Dr. Klaus Boller p7bl, ©Eye of Science p7cr, ©Michael Abbey p7br, ©Kenneth Eward/BioGrafx p17c.

All rights reserved under the International and Pan-American Copyright Convention. No part of this publication may be reproduced, stored in a retrieval system or transmitted in any form or by any means, electronic, mechanical, photocopying, recording or otherwise, without the prior written permission of the copyright owners. Published in the United States by Frederic Thomas Inc.

Printed in U.S.A. All rights reserved.

FREDERIC THOMAS INC.

Produced by Frederic Thomas Inc., Naples, Florida, Tel: 239-593-8000

Clean Kids, Happy Kids

Written by Jean Fischer

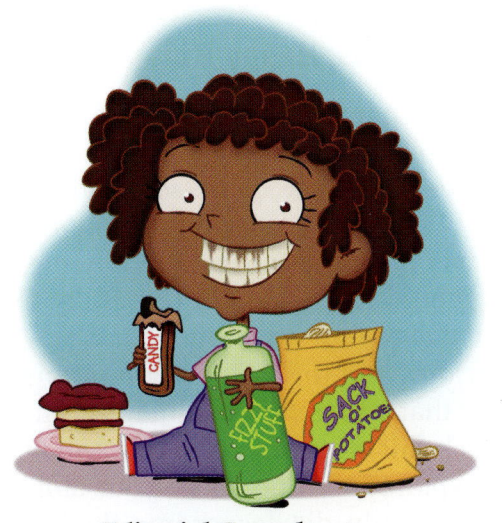

Editorial Consultant
American School Health Association

ASHA

"Kid's Health is our First Priority."

Creative Director Tom Gawle
Senior Editor Mary Weber
Designers Tim Carls and Mike Hopkins
Photographers Saturn Lounge and Clic Photography
Illustrators Maggie Downer, Jim Durk, Ken Edwards,
Steve Haefele, Joe Mathieu, Jesus Redondo,
Robert Roper, Studio Ferrer and Thompson Bros.

Special thanks to our Growing & Going™ Kids
Andrea, Becky, Garrett, Isabella, Justin,
Kaitlyn, Kristina, Nina, Shane and Travis

Parent Note: Clean Kids, Happy Kids

As parents, you are obviously concerned about your children's health, fitness and safety. You want to ensure that they have all the information they need to grow up fit, safe and well. This is where the *Growing & Going*™ series can help. By reading these books together as a family, you will have peace of mind knowing that your children understand the importance of getting physically fit, staying healthy and being safe in day-to-day situations.

Kids are curious, and the information in this series is sure to prompt questions that you and your children can examine together. Each book is chock full of information that can be used as a springboard for exploration. Encourage your children to question and explore. Then, as a family, dig deeper into the issues, and make healthy living a priority in your household.

In this book, *Clean Kids, Happy Kids*, your children will discover dozens of helpful facts about health and personal hygiene. They will learn about germs and how to keep them from spreading around. They will find out the best ways to care for their teeth and what to expect at a routine visit to a pediatrician. And, before they are through, they will know just what to do to keep their bodies neat and clean.

Along with integrating the information in the *Growing & Going* series into your family's daily lifestyle, we also recommend that you complete a CPR course. Many hospitals and health organizations offer first-aid and safety classes designed to help parents and caregivers cope with emergency situations, and keep the home environment safe for children.

Clean Up and Be Happy

It feels good to be clean and healthy. In fact, being clean and healthy makes you a happier kid. Get together with your family and friends and discuss these questions. See how much you know about being clean and healthy.

1. When should you wash your hands?
2. How often should you brush your teeth?
3. Can you list five healthy foods? Explain why they're healthy.
4. How are colds spread?
5. How often should you exercise?
6. Why is it important to bathe often?

If you don't know the answers to all of these questions, that's okay. By the time you've finished reading *Clean Kids, Happy Kids*, you'll know all about looking and feeling great. When you're done with the book, come back to this page. See if you would answer the questions differently and then take the Clean Kids Challenge on pages 30-31.

Note to Kids

You are in charge of your body. It is yours to keep for the rest of your life. So you want to take really good care of it. All through this book you will find Rickey, who is a very helpful raccoon. Rickey likes to hang out with kids, is very bright and will tell you lots of neat stuff about staying healthy and clean. Along the way there will be fun things to do and things to learn that you can share with your friends.

Did you know that billions of germs are living on your body – right now? You'll learn about germs in this book. You'll find out what teeth are made of and how they help you to talk. And if you've ever wondered why people sweat and what sweat is made of, that's in here, too!

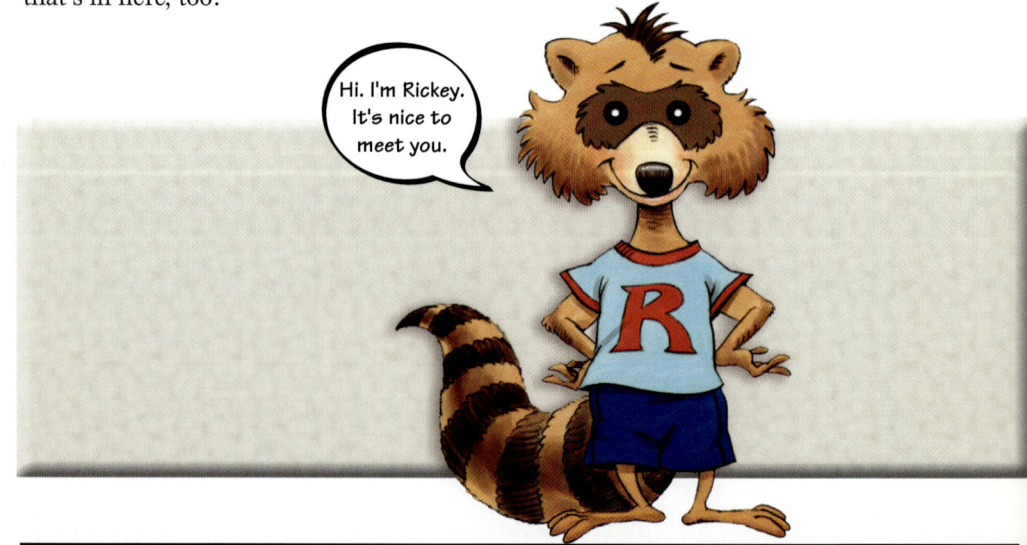

The Truth About Germs

The bacteria in the mouth help break down the food you eat. Without helpful bacteria, you would starve. But some bacteria can cause illness. The bacteria, viruses and other tiny organisms that can make people sick are germs. You have billions of them hanging out all over your body – on your hair, under your fingernails and on your skin. Eeeeeewwwww! They are small and sneaky. These pictures below were taken through a microscope. But don't worry, there are ways you can keep germs from making you sick. There are four germ families. Let's find out what they're up to.

Meet the Bacteria Family

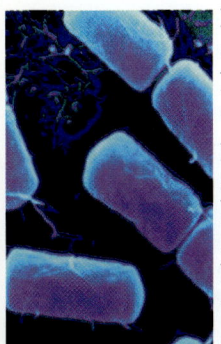

Bacteria (back-teer-ea) can cause nasty things like infections, toothaches and pneumonia. They do good things, too. Some live in your stomach and intestines. They help break down the food you eat so nutrients can nourish your body.

Meet the Fungi Family

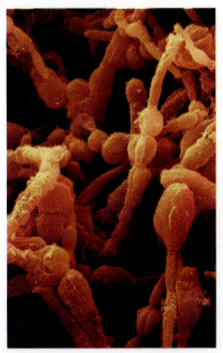

Members of the **Fungi** (fun-guy) family are plant-like germs that hang out in warm, damp places. They can cause diseases like athlete's foot and ringworm. They usually aren't dangerous, but they're not fun either.

Meet the Virus Family

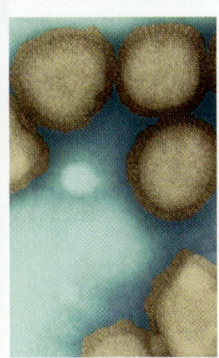

The **Virus** (vi-rus) family includes germs that cause colds, chickenpox and flu. They hang out in the air and on surfaces like pencils, disks and hands. When you sneeze, viruses spray out of your mouth and land everywhere. They love to travel.

Meet the Protozoa Family

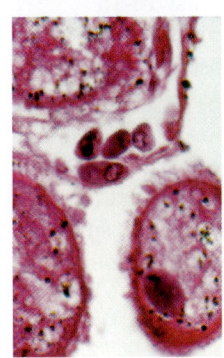

Protozoa (pro-toe-zoh-a) are tiny one-celled animals that like moist places. In fact, you can often find the protozoans in water that is not purified. If you get an upset stomach and diarrhea, a protozoan might be the culprit.

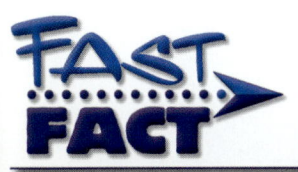

FAST FACT

The U.S. Centers for Disease Control says that hand washing is one of the best ways to stop the spread of illnesses like colds, flu and diarrhea.

7

Start with Your Hands

Germs can enter your body when your unwashed hands touch your nose, mouth or open cuts. So, to keep that from happening, wash your hands often.

How to Wash Your Hands

Don't just swish your hands with soap and water and say that you're done. That's like giving germs a quick zap with a squirt gun. What you want to do is give those germs a bath that they'll never forget!

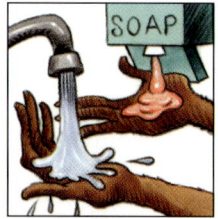

1. Wet your hands. Use soap and running water to make lather – or lots of bubbles.

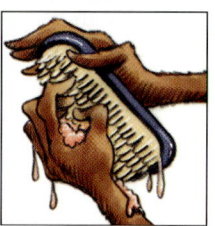

2. Wash your hands front and back, top and bottom and between the fingers. Scrub your wrists and fingernails with a brush.

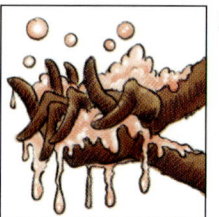

3. Rub your soapy hands together for at least 10-15 seconds. Shake those germs loose!

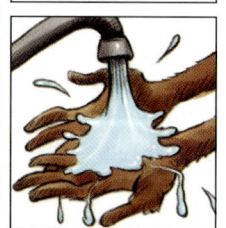

4. Rinse your hands well, and let those dirty germs spin down the drain.

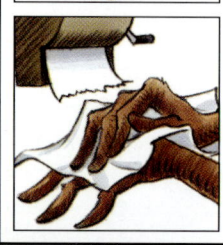

5. Dry your hands with a paper towel or clean towel.

When to Wash Your Hands

Wash your hands before you:
- eat or prepare food.
- help someone who is sick or hurt.
- touch a cut or sore.
- put in or take out contact lenses.

Wash your hands after you:
- sneeze, cough or blow your nose.
- go to the bathroom.
- change a baby's diaper.
- handle uncooked meat.
- touch garbage.
- touch an animal.
- get rid of animal poop.
- help someone who is sick or hurt.
- touch a cut or sore.

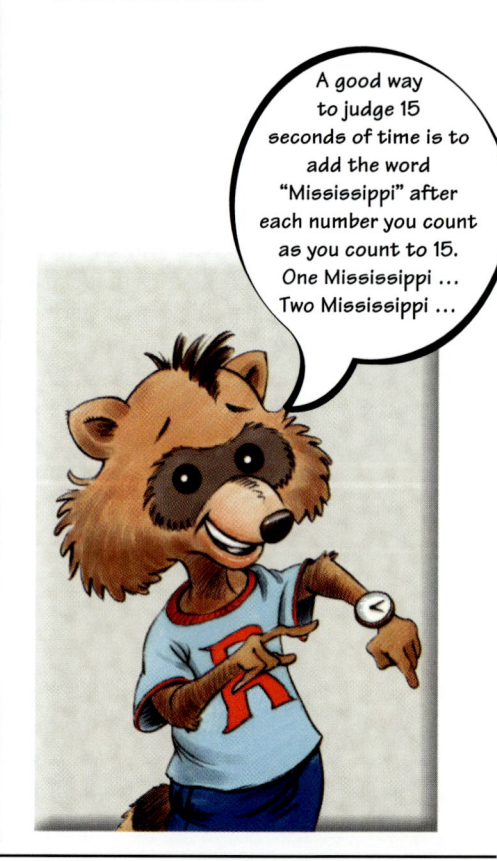

A good way to judge 15 seconds of time is to add the word "Mississippi" after each number you count as you count to 15. One Mississippi … Two Mississippi …

Nails – Fingers and Toes

The space between your nails and skin is a favorite hiding place for all kinds of germs. If you have dirt under your fingernails and you touch your mouth, you could even eat germs. Anything you touch that isn't clean can end up stuck under your nails, or worse – in you.

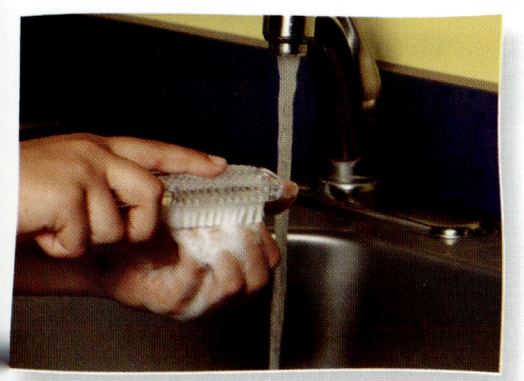

How Fast Do Nails Grow?

Nails grow at different rates in different people. The average nail grows one-eighth inch per month, which means that it usually takes between four and six months to grow a whole new nail. Fingernails grow faster on young people, boys and in the summer. Toenails grow much more slowly.

Toenail clippers are larger than fingernail clippers and snip the toenail straight across. This helps prevent ingrown toenails, which can be painful.

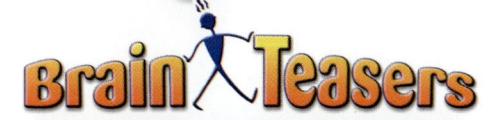

Clean Your Nails

When you wash your hands, clean under your nails using plenty of soap and water. If they're really dirty, use a nailbrush or an old toothbrush to get the dirt out from under them. Wash the dirt away with lots of water. When you take a bath or shower, don't forget to wash under your toenails, too. Your nails should be clipped short and without any ragged or sharp edges. You may need a parent's help with this.

WHY DO ELEPHANTS PAINT THEIR TOENAILS RED?

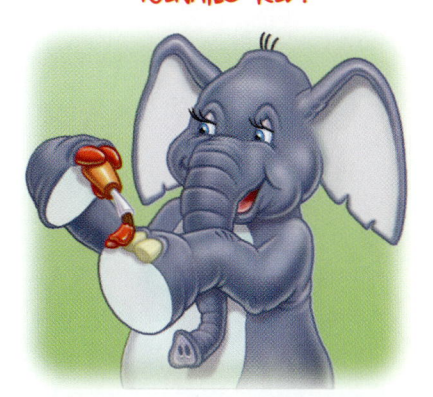

Answer: So they can hide in the branches of cherry trees.

Brain Teasers

Just How Fast Do Your Nails Grow?

Measure each toenail and fingernail. Measure the length of your nails from the base to the tip each week. Ask a parent, brother or sister to do the same. Record the results on a chart to keep track. What differences do you see? Do fingernails grow faster than toenails? Does one nail grow faster than all others? Whose nails grow the fastest?

9

Talking Through Your Teeth

Do you know that teeth help you to speak? Say the word "tooth." Your tongue brushes across your top teeth to make the "th" sound. Besides helping you to speak, teeth help you to look good. Without them, the muscles around your mouth would sag inward, your lips would look thin and your cheeks would cave in!

What Is a Tooth Made Of?

The part of the tooth that appears above the **gums** is called a **crown**. The tops of some crowns have little "waves" called **cusps**. Crowns are covered with a thin layer of **enamel,** made mostly of minerals and just a little water. It makes your teeth look white, and it is the hardest tissue in your body.

Inside a tooth, the innermost layer is called **pulp**. It includes **blood vessels** to nourish the tooth and **nerves** to send messages to the brain. When you have a toothache, these nerves tell your brain, "Ouch!"

Between pulp and enamel is a yellowish layer called **dentin**. It's harder than bone and is made mostly of minerals and water.

The tooth part below the gums is called a **root.** It and the surrounding **tissue** hold a tooth firmly inside your **jaw**. Otherwise, it would fall out!

The top layer of a root is called **cementum.** This layer is also made of minerals and water, but it's not quite as hard as bone or enamel.

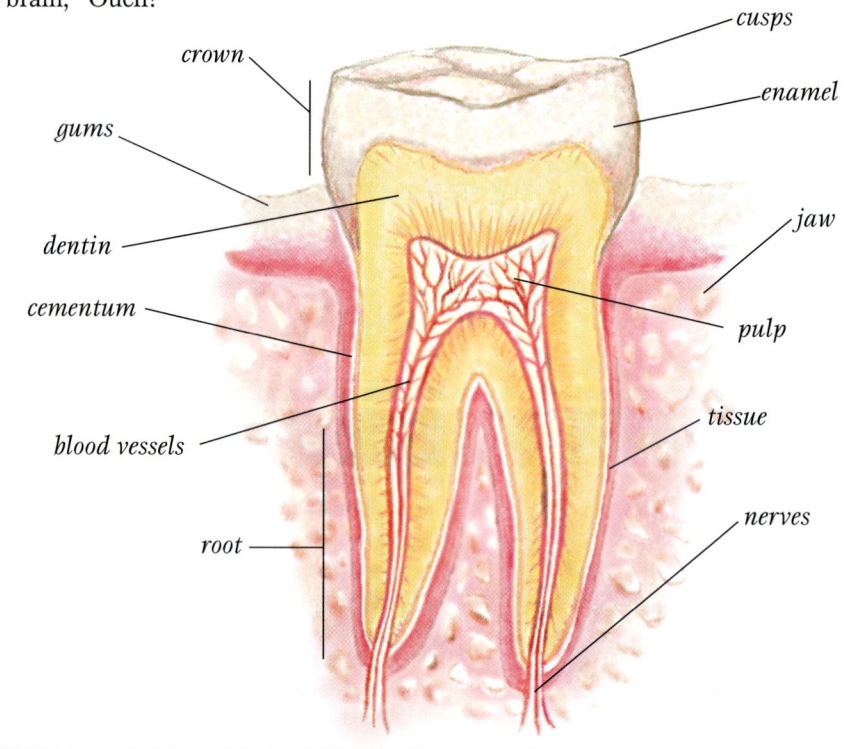

The Anatomy of a Cavity

STEP 1. Kid eats foods high in sugar and starch, like soda, cake, crackers, cereal and candy.

STEP 2. Kid doesn't clean teeth often enough or well enough, leaving small bits of food on and in between teeth.

STEP 3. Bacteria that live in the mouth eat the bits of food left on the teeth. When bacteria eat, they produce acid. Over time, the acid starts to destroy the protective enamel on the teeth. That's how Kid gets cavities!

What holds those pesky bacteria and the acid onto your teeth? How come they don't just get washed off and swallowed? The answer is **plaque** (plack) – a clear film of saliva and food particles that sticks to your teeth. Plaque acts like a magnet for bacteria and for sugar. Plaque also holds the acid and keeps it close to the tooth's enamel, and that leads to cavities.

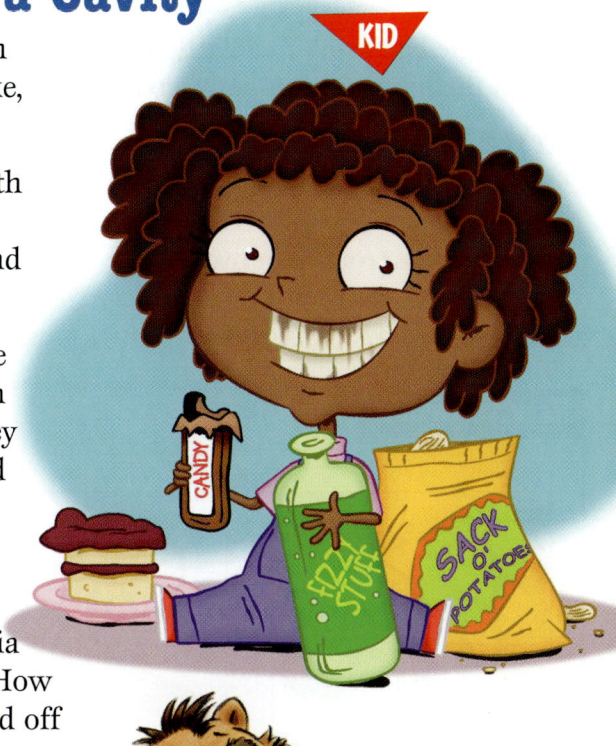

Hmmmm. This isn't good.

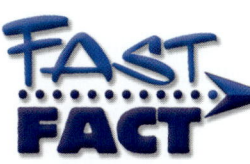

FAST FACT

Since way back in 1946, communities all across America have added fluoride to their drinking water. Many people believe that fluoride helps prevent tooth decay. Fluoride is a mineral that is found naturally in water. Researchers have found that it makes teeth stronger and more resistant to acid. Not everyone agrees about how much fluoride is best for kids. So, to be on the safe side, ask your dentist for advice.

The War Against Tooth Decay

Let's battle bacteria! The battle plans on pages 12 through 17 will give you all the ammunition you need to win the war against tooth decay.

BATTLE PLAN A: Brush and Floss

According to the American Dental Association, you should brush your teeth twice a day using a soft-bristled brush. Once a day, use dental floss to remove plaque from in between teeth. Brushing and flossing are the best things you can do to prevent cavities. You should have your own toothbrush, and replace it every 3 to 4 months. Toothbrushes wear out.

How to Brush

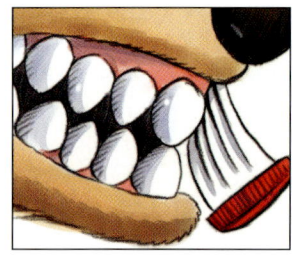

1. Place the toothbrush bristles at a 45-degree angle where your teeth meet your gums.

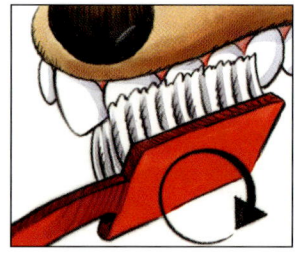

2. Gently move it back and forth in short, circular strokes as wide as the tooth you are brushing.

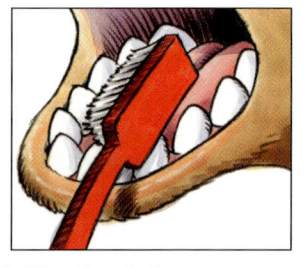

3. First brush the outer surfaces of your teeth, then the inner surfaces and finally the chewing surfaces.

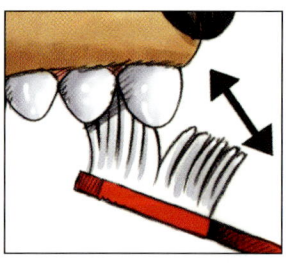

4. Using the tip of the brush, clean the inside of your front teeth. This time use gentle up-and-down strokes.

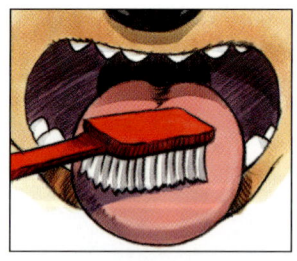

5. The last thing to do is brush your tongue, just in case any bacteria are hanging out on it.

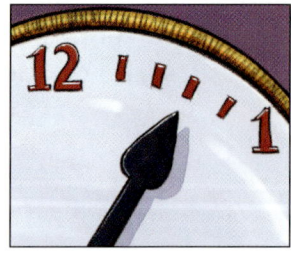

6. Don't be in a hurry. It takes 2-3 minutes to do a good job of tooth brushing.

Are You Bored with Your Toothbrush?

Modern toothbrushes come in all sorts of colors and designs. The early Chinese people invented what may have been the first brush to be used on teeth. The bristles were made of hairs from the neck of the Siberian boar! In fact, animal hair was used to make toothbrushes all the way up to 1937, when nylon was invented by Wallace H. Carothers in the U.S.A.

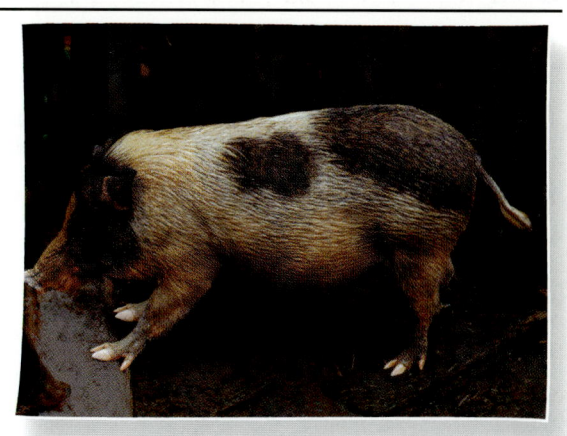

How to Floss

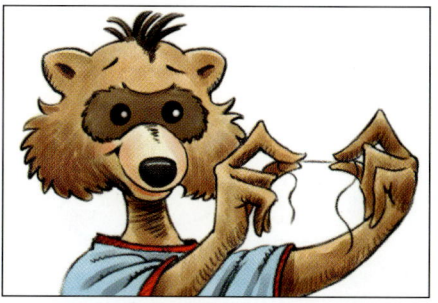

1. Hold a piece of dental floss tightly between your thumbs and forefingers.

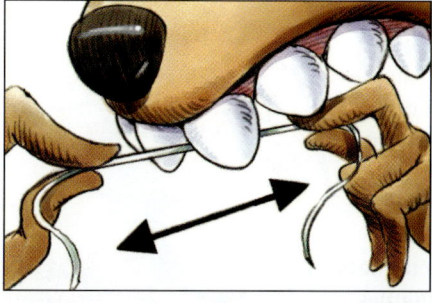

2. Slide it between two teeth and begin moving it in a gentle rubbing motion, working from the top down. Do not floss into the gums.

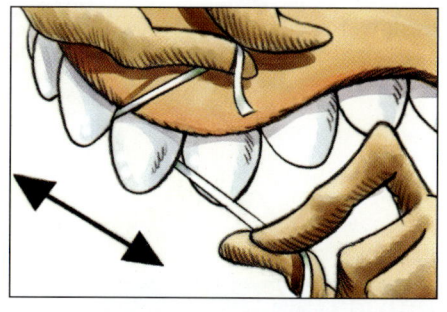

3. When the floss gets to the gum line, curve it into a C shape against one tooth. Then carefully slide it into the space between the gum and the tooth. Gently rub the sides of the tooth, using an up and down motion. Then bend it around the next tooth.

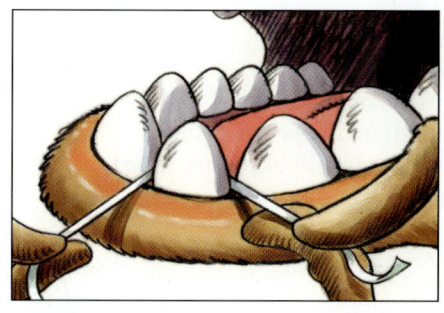

4. Repeat this action for each tooth until you've done them all.

The Food You Chew!

Every time you eat something that contains sugar or starch, bacteria can attack your teeth for 20 minutes or more! There are certain types of food that they like and others that they dislike. And guess what – you're the one who decides what they eat!

BATTLE PLAN B: Eat Smart

Rule number one: avoid sticky, gooey and chewy foods. They hang onto teeth and make a feast for bacteria. Eat smart by choosing a variety of foods from the following list.

Fresh Fruits and Raw Vegetables

berries
ora**n**ges
grapefruit
mel**o**ns
pineapple
pears
tangerines
bro**c**coli
celery
carrots
cucumbers
tomatoes
unsweetened fruit and
vegetable juices

Grains

bread
plain bagels
unsweetened cereals
unbuttered popcorn
tort**i**lla chips (baked, not fried)
pasta

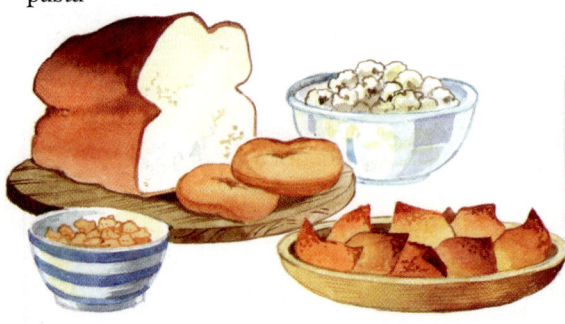

Milk and Dairy Products

low- or non-fat milk
low- or non-fa**t** yogurt
low- or non-fat cheeses
low- or non-fat cottage cheese

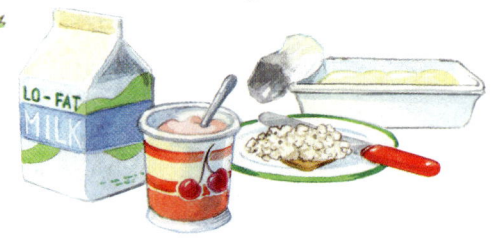

Meat, Nuts and Seeds

ch**i**cken
turkey
sliced meats
pumpkin seeds
sunflower s**e**eds
nut**s**

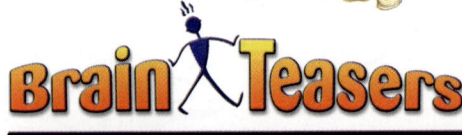

Brain Teasers

A Special Message from All the Food Groups

For a special message, print in order on the lines below all the bold letters found, top to bottom, on the food list above.

_____ _____

Answer: no cavities

The Truth About Snacks

Many kids (and grownups, too) like to snack on things that have sugar and starch (like candy, cookies and potato chips). You already know that these things are bad for your teeth. When you eat sticky, gooey or chewy snacks, the food stays in your mouth longer. So, if you snack at all, choose smart snacks like raw veggies, or fruit.

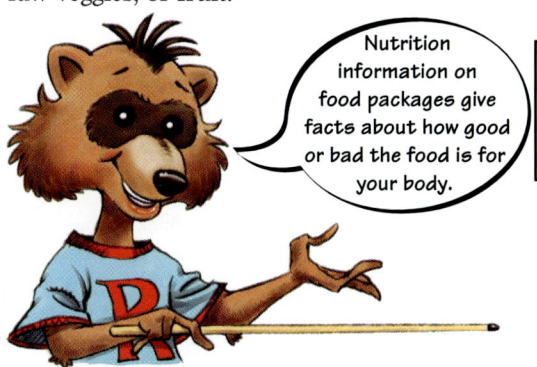

Nutrition information on food packages give facts about how good or bad the food is for your body.

Hanging Out with Sugar and Goo

When your grandparents were kids, people didn't know as much about tooth care as they do today. Kids back then hung out at **soda fountains** – restaurants that sold mostly sugary treats. They ate gooey ice-cream treats and fizzy sugar-filled sodas. No wonder kids had more cavities back in the 1950s.

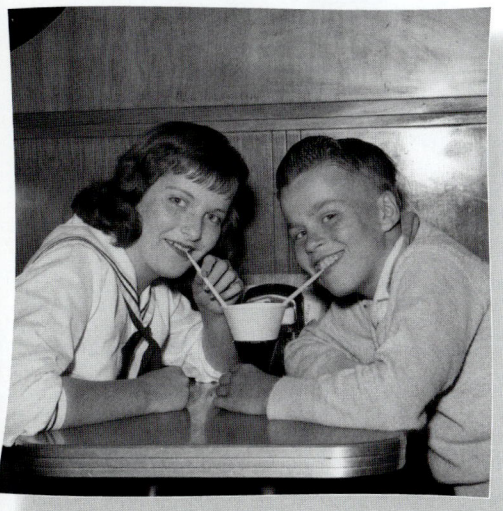

Maps to Smart Eating

Labels on food packages list what's in the food – the ingredients. Look for foods low in sugar and fat. These foods won't give bacteria much to eat. Foods high in calcium are good for your teeth, too. Calcium is a mineral the body uses to make dentin, enamel and cementum.

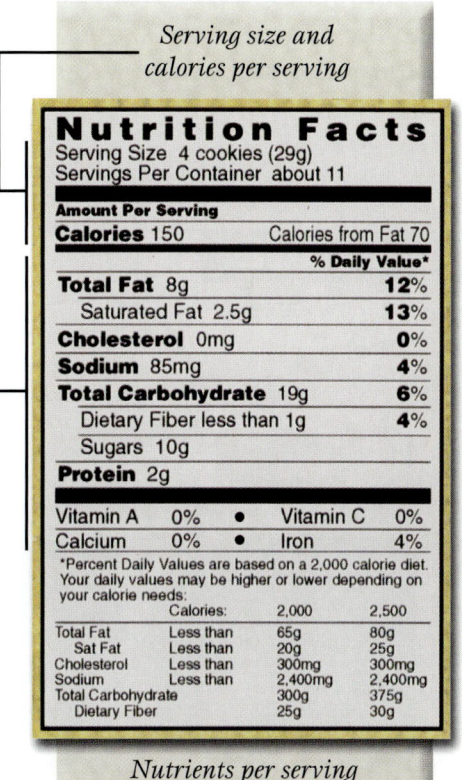

Serving size and calories per serving

Nutrition Facts
Serving Size 4 cookies (29g)
Servings Per Container about 11

Amount Per Serving	
Calories 150	Calories from Fat 70
	% Daily Value*
Total Fat 8g	12%
Saturated Fat 2.5g	13%
Cholesterol 0mg	0%
Sodium 85mg	4%
Total Carbohydrate 19g	6%
Dietary Fiber less than 1g	4%
Sugars 10g	
Protein 2g	

| Vitamin A | 0% | • | Vitamin C | 0% |
| Calcium | 0% | • | Iron | 4% |

*Percent Daily Values are based on a 2,000 calorie diet. Your daily values may be higher or lower depending on your calorie needs:

		Calories:	2,000	2,500
Total Fat	Less than		65g	80g
Sat Fat	Less than		20g	25g
Cholesterol	Less than		300mg	300mg
Sodium	Less than		2,400mg	2,400mg
Total Carbohydrate			300g	375g
Dietary Fiber			25g	30g

Nutrients per serving including starches, sugars (carbohydrates) and calcium

These foods are high in calcium. Try one the next time you want a snack.

- cheese
- yogurt
- almonds
- milk
- beans
- spinach
- rhubarb
- grilled cheese sandwich
- macaroni and cheese
- dark green leafy veggies
- pudding
- creamed soups
- milk-based chowders
- bok choy

15

The Dentist Is In

Even if you do a great job taking care of your teeth by brushing, flossing and eating right, you might still get cavities. Enlist the help of your dentist.

BATTLE PLAN C: Make Regular Visits to the Dentist

Why is a dentist your best buddy in the war against tooth decay? Because he or she is a doctor specially trained to care for your teeth. According to the American Academy of Pediatric Dentistry, you should go to the dentist every six months for a cleaning and checkup. If you have cavities or anything else wrong with your teeth, your dentist will know what to do.

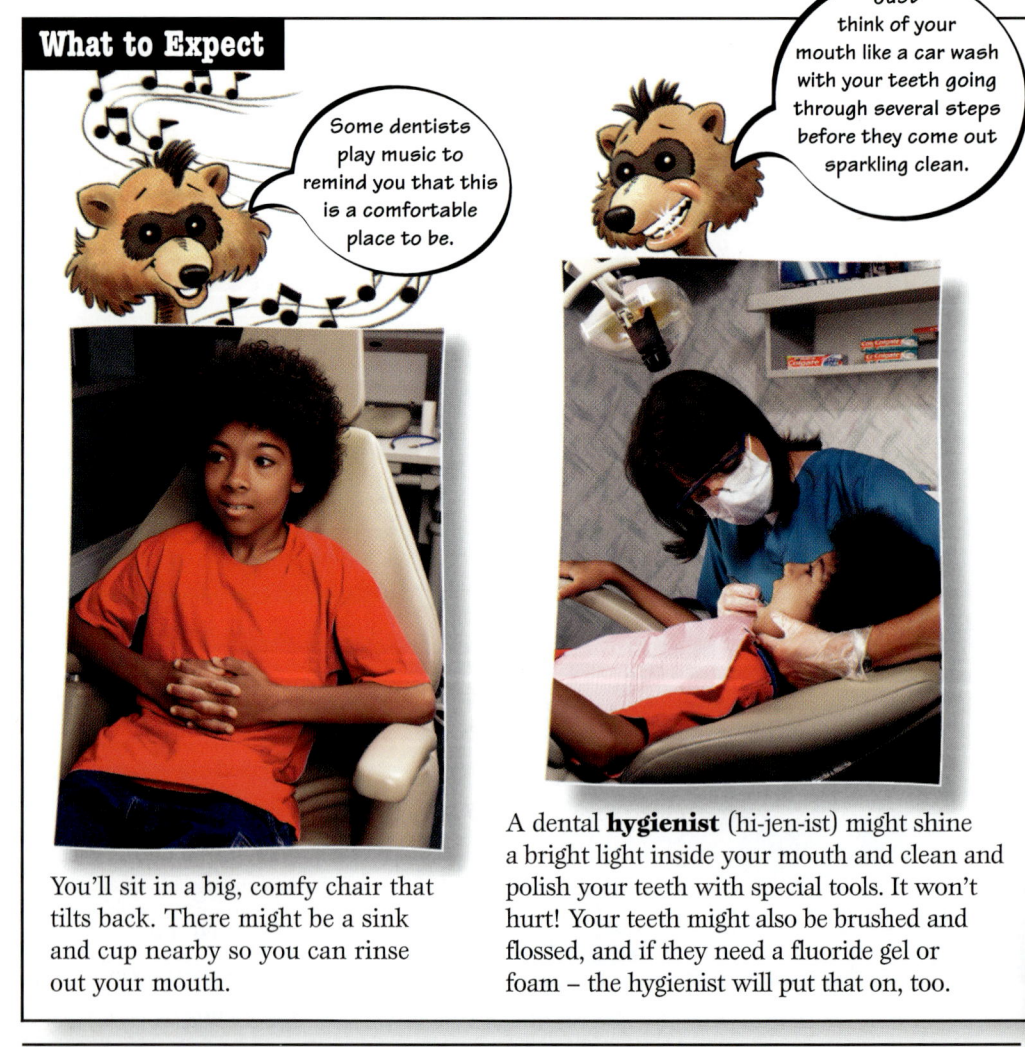

What to Expect

Some dentists play music to remind you that this is a comfortable place to be.

Just think of your mouth like a car wash with your teeth going through several steps before they come out sparkling clean.

You'll sit in a big, comfy chair that tilts back. There might be a sink and cup nearby so you can rinse out your mouth.

A dental **hygienist** (hi-jen-ist) might shine a bright light inside your mouth and clean and polish your teeth with special tools. It won't hurt! Your teeth might also be brushed and flossed, and if they need a fluoride gel or foam – the hygienist will put that on, too.

Brain Teasers

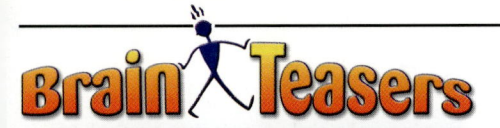

About Your Teeth

1. Which one of these snacks will keep your teeth strong and healthy?
   a. candy bar
   b. can of soda
   c. licorice stick
   d. none of the above

2. Calcium is a mineral that helps make strong bones and teeth and is found in_____.
   a. milk
   b. almonds
   c. dark green leafy vegetables
   d. all of the above

3. A toothbrush will wear out from use. You should get a new one every 3-4 months.
   a. true
   b. false

4. How often should you have a dental checkup?
   a. once a month
   b. when you turn 16 years old
   c. every six months
   d. all of the above

5. You should brush your teeth_____.
   a. twice a day
   b. with a soft-bristle toothbrush
   c. to prevent the build up of plaque
   d. all of the above

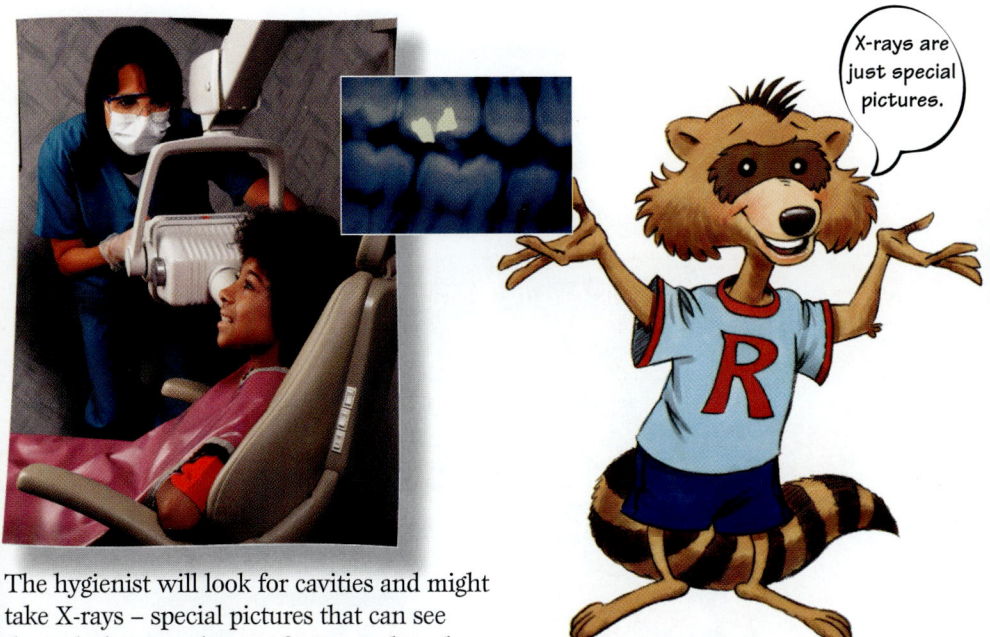

Answers: 1. d; 2. d; 3. a; 4. c; 5. d

X-rays are just special pictures.

The hygienist will look for cavities and might take X-rays – special pictures that can see through the outer layers of your teeth and below the gums.

The dentist will look at the X-rays to see if you have cavities or gum problems and see if your teeth are coming in straight and strong. If they aren't coming in right, the dentist might want you to see an **orthodontist** (or-tho-don-tist), a doctor who helps straighten teeth with braces.

Fix Those Cavities!
To fix a cavity, a dentist gives you medicine to numb the nerves around the tooth so it won't hurt. Then, using special tools, he or she removes the decayed part and fills your tooth with a special material to make it strong and healthy again. That's it, you're done!

Eat Right and Feel Good

Are you the kind of kid who trades a nutritious lunch for a bag of chips and a brownie? Once in a while, a few chips or a brownie is a nice treat, but you can't live on them. Not getting exercise and eating poorly will make your body a campground for germs. If your body isn't fit and strong, it won't be able to put up a good fight against viruses and other germs. That means that you could get sick more often and stay sick longer. So, what can you do about it? Let's find out.

The Food Guide Pyramid

The Food Guide Pyramid is a guide to healthy eating. It shows the groups of food you need to eat each day, and how much. Do you see that the pyramid is getting skinnier toward the top? That tells you not to eat much of these foods. The groups at the bottom are foods you can eat more of. As you climb the pyramid, you'll find foods that you should eat less often. The foods at the very top are high in fat and have added sugar. They should be eaten least of all.

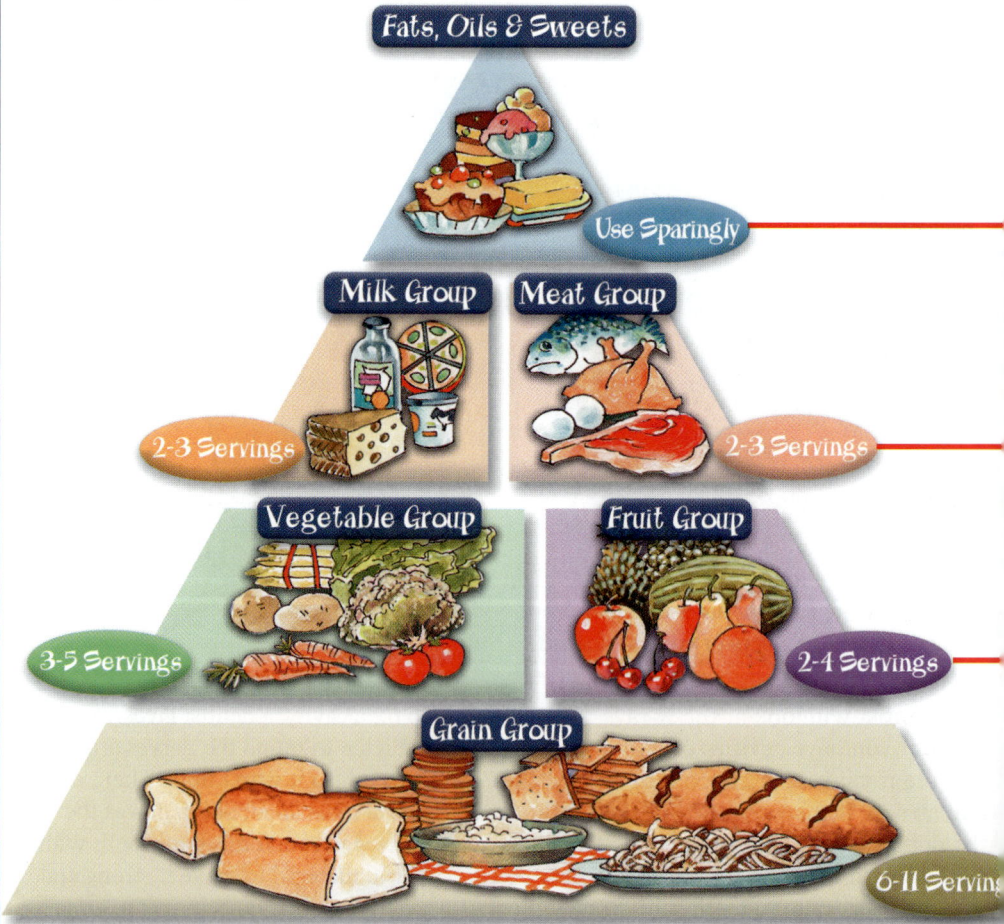

Fats, Oils & Sweets — Use Sparingly

Milk Group — 2-3 Servings

Meat Group — 2-3 Servings

Vegetable Group — 3-5 Servings

Fruit Group — 2-4 Servings

Grain Group — 6-11 Servings

Wash Your Fruits and Veggies

You earn extra clean-kid points if you wash your hands, then peel or wash your fruits and veggies before you eat them. Why? Because washing them under cold, running water will rinse away any bacteria that are hanging out on them. Better down the drain than inside of you! And don't use soap or detergent when you wash fruits and veggies. That will make them taste bad.

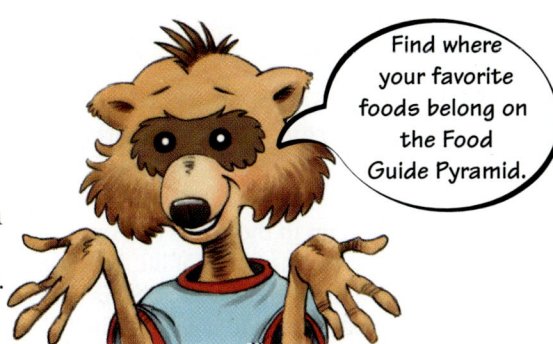

How Much Do You Need?

The U.S. Department of Agriculture suggests a certain number of servings for each food group on the pyramid. That's how many servings you should have each day. A serving size depends on things like your age, weight and health. Ask your doctor to suggest serving sizes the next time you go for a checkup.

Level Four: Sugar and fat are at the top – things like candy, cookies, sugary sodas and high-fat chips. They provide energy and fat, but not much else. Eat very little of these.

Level Three: These foods – dairy products, meats, beans, fish, eggs and nuts – have calcium, protein and some vitamins, minerals and fat. You need some, but not a lot of these, every day. Peanut butter and cheese are in this group.

Level Two: Fruits and vegetables are here with many vitamins and minerals that our bodies need as well as energy. 100% fruit juice, beans, peas and bananas are some of the foods on this level.

Level One: At the bottom are bread, cereal, rice and pasta. These foods give you energy and some vitamins and minerals. Toast, cold cereal and macaroni fall into this group.

Find where your favorite foods belong on the Food Guide Pyramid.

Brain Teasers

Are You Food Smart?

Each food listed below has a box next to it. Write the correct Food Pyramid Level (1-4) number in the box. The first one is done for you.

- [4] 1. Doughnut
- [ ] 2. Orange soda
- [ ] 3. Watermelon
- [ ] 4. Chocolate bar
- [ ] 5. Bagel
- [ ] 6. Cottage cheese
- [ ] 7. Ice cream
- [ ] 8. Kiwi
- [ ] 9. Chicken breast
- [ ] 10. Saltine cracker
- [ ] 11. Lima beans
- [ ] 12. Pistachio nuts
- [ ] 13. Peas
- [ ] 14. Plum
- [ ] 15. Oatmeal

Answers: Doughnut 4, Orange soda 4, Watermelon 2, Chocolate bar 4, Bagel 1, Cottage cheese 3, Ice cream 4, Kiwi 2, Chicken breast 3, Saltine cracker 1, Lima beans 2, Pistachio nuts 3, Peas 2, Plum 2, Oatmeal 1.

Don't Just Sit There

Now that you know all about eating foods that keep you healthy, strong and full of energy, there is another pyramid to help you have fun and stay physically fit.

If you had grown up in the 1800s on America's Great Plains, you wouldn't have thought about exercising. Exercise was a way of life. In those days, kids walked or rode horses wherever they went because there were no bikes or cars. Kids gardened, milked cows, gathered eggs, cleaned out barns, hauled water and helped in the fields. A kid's life on the prairie was filled with activity. There were no televisions, no computers – and no couch potatoes!

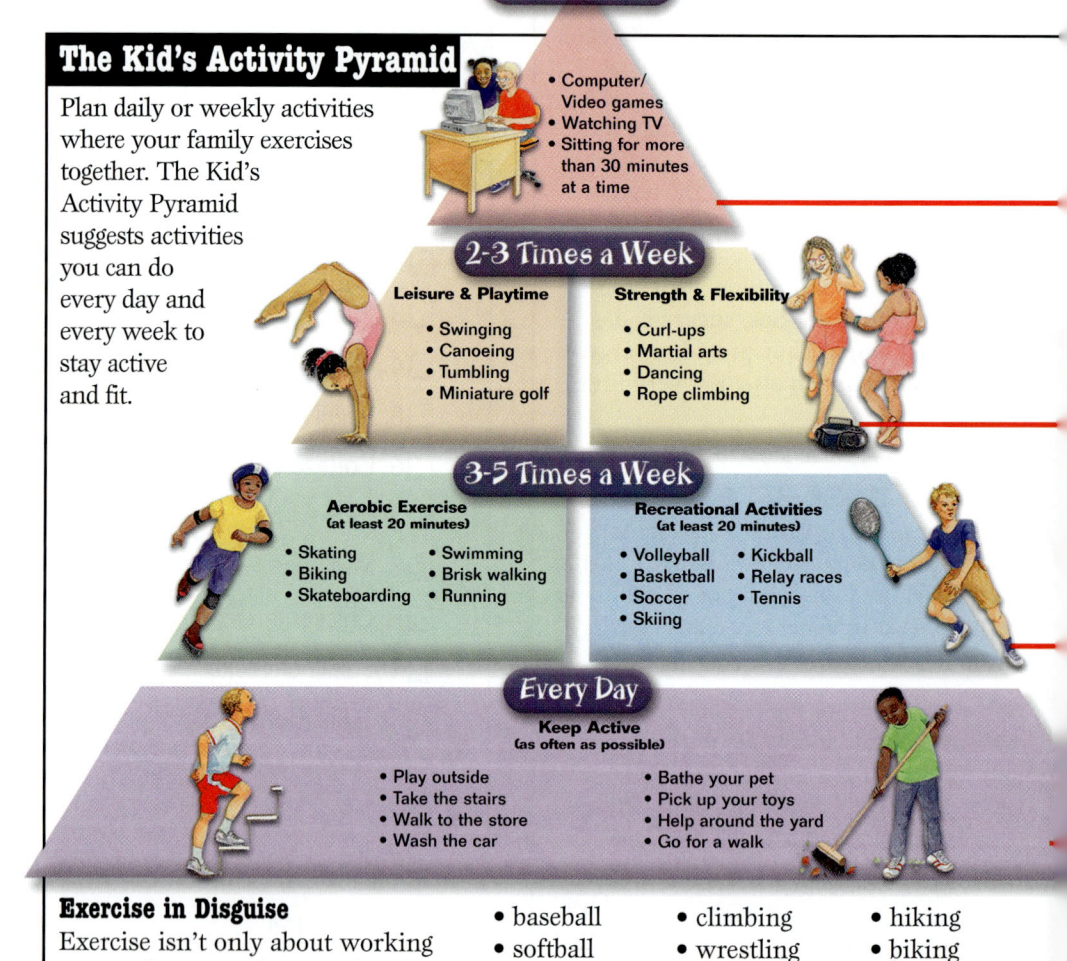

The Kid's Activity Pyramid

Plan daily or weekly activities where your family exercises together. The Kid's Activity Pyramid suggests activities you can do every day and every week to stay active and fit.

Cut Down On
- Computer/Video games
- Watching TV
- Sitting for more than 30 minutes at a time

2-3 Times a Week

Leisure & Playtime
- Swinging
- Canoeing
- Tumbling
- Miniature golf

Strength & Flexibility
- Curl-ups
- Martial arts
- Dancing
- Rope climbing

3-5 Times a Week

Aerobic Exercise (at least 20 minutes)
- Skating
- Biking
- Skateboarding
- Swimming
- Brisk walking
- Running

Recreational Activities (at least 20 minutes)
- Volleyball
- Basketball
- Soccer
- Skiing
- Kickball
- Relay races
- Tennis

Every Day

Keep Active (as often as possible)
- Play outside
- Take the stairs
- Walk to the store
- Wash the car
- Bathe your pet
- Pick up your toys
- Help around the yard
- Go for a walk

Exercise in Disguise

Exercise isn't only about working out, push-ups, pull-ups and jumping up and down. It's about having fun! Physical fitness is hiding in each of these sports and activities.

- baseball
- softball
- football
- basketball
- hockey
- soccer
- climbing
- wrestling
- karate
- tennis
- swimming
- skating
- hiking
- biking
- dancing
- jump rope
- gardening
- skateboarding

KID

Are You a Couch Potato?
According to the President's Council on Physical Fitness and Sports, one of every four kids in the U.S.A. spends four hours or more watching television each day. Are you one of them? If you are, turn off the TV and do something!

Make It a Family Affair
Think of ways that your family can exercise together. Then plan to make it a daily or weekly activity. You can take a walk, bike, play softball or go swimming. Think of yourself as a coach. Can you whip your family into shape and get them physically fit?

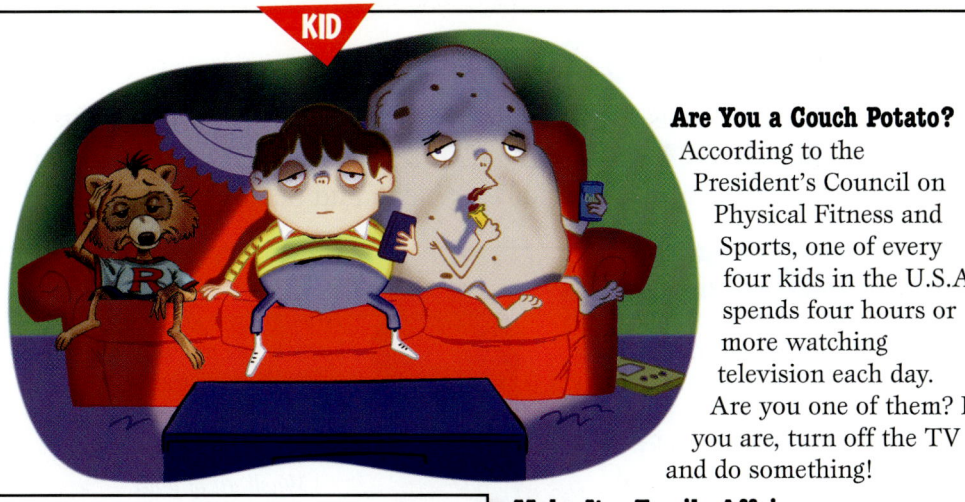

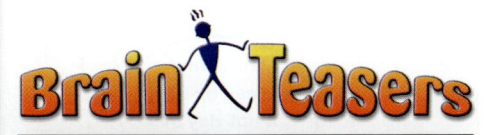

Level Four: Visit the top of the pyramid anytime after exercising at level 1, 2 or 3. This is where you can rest, watch TV, use the computer or play video games. But don't stay here! You need to climb the pyramid every day.

Level Three: This is where you build strong muscles with activities like push-ups, pull-ups, climbing ropes, swinging on a swing, dancing or hiking. Find activities that you like. That way, you'll keep on doing them.

Level Two: These are the aerobic exercises – like swimming, basketball, biking and tennis. They keep your heart and lungs healthy and strong and build strength and endurance.

Level One: The bottom of the pyramid is the base. If you're not an active kid, or if you're overweight, do "base" activities until your body doesn't get tired doing them. Move up the pyramid when you feel ready. If it takes a while to move up, don't feel bad. Many kids are just like you. You can do it; don't give up!

Brain Teasers
Words That Get You Moving
How many other ways can you think of to get some exercise? Here's a game to try. Think of action words – verbs – that describe something active that you do. Words like run, jump, race and slide. Now add to the list. How many action words can you think of?

_____   _____
_____   _____
_____   _____
_____   _____
_____   _____
_____   _____
_____   _____
_____   _____
_____   _____

Skin Holds You In

Do you know that skin is the largest organ of your body? Skin also lets you feel things – heat, cold, hard, soft. And since skin is a part of you that other people see, you'll want to keep it looking clean and healthy all the time.

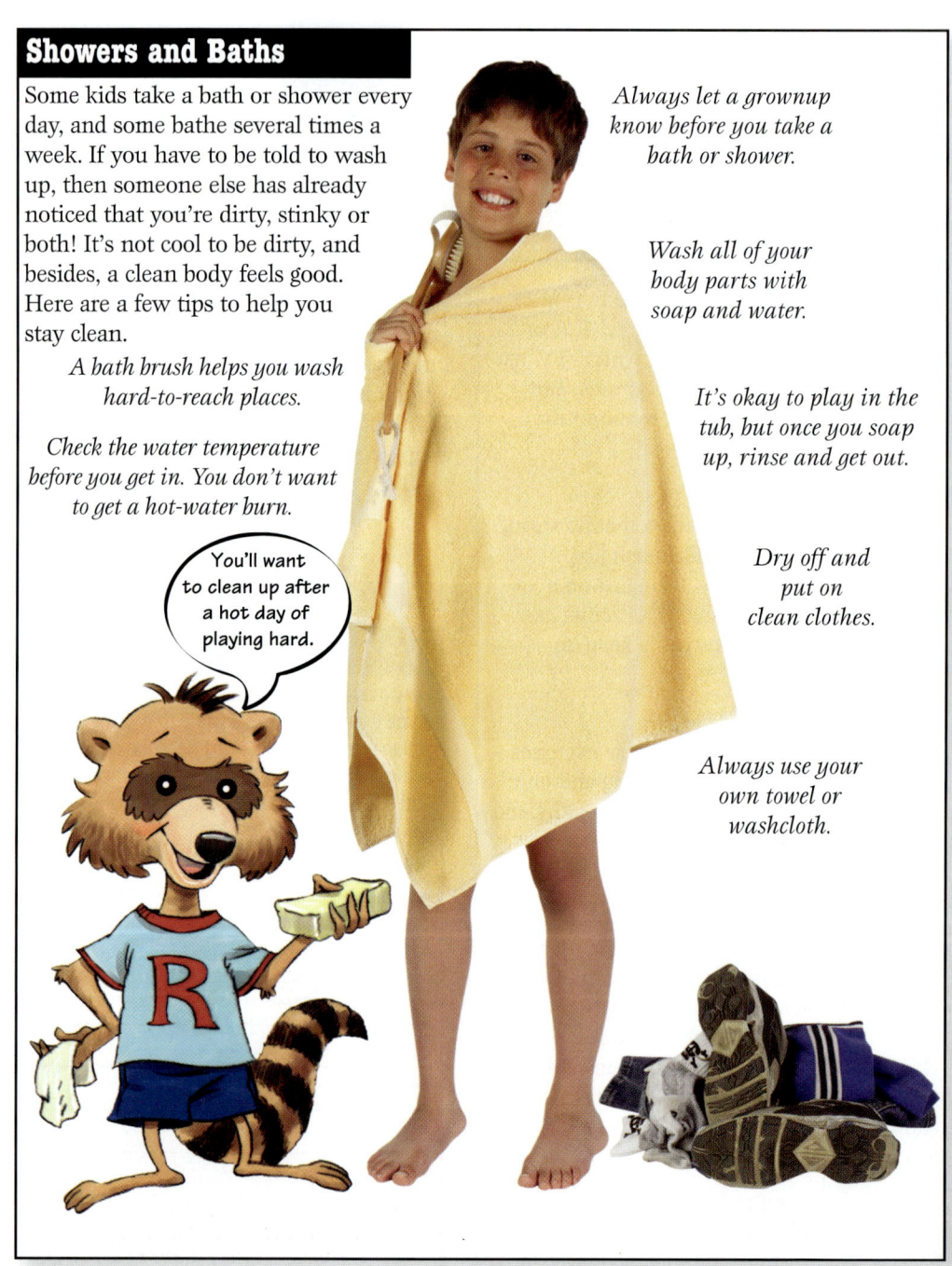

Showers and Baths

Some kids take a bath or shower every day, and some bathe several times a week. If you have to be told to wash up, then someone else has already noticed that you're dirty, stinky or both! It's not cool to be dirty, and besides, a clean body feels good. Here are a few tips to help you stay clean.

A bath brush helps you wash hard-to-reach places.

Check the water temperature before you get in. You don't want to get a hot-water burn.

Always let a grownup know before you take a bath or shower.

Wash all of your body parts with soap and water.

It's okay to play in the tub, but once you soap up, rinse and get out.

Dry off and put on clean clothes.

Always use your own towel or washcloth.

You'll want to clean up after a hot day of playing hard.

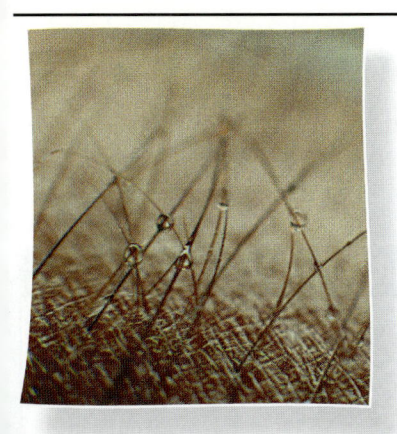

The Truth About Sweat

Sweat glands in your skin make sweat. Sweat is made mostly of water, minerals and a few other things. It leaves your body through tiny holes in your skin, called **pores.** Sweat is a liquid, and when it hits the air it evaporates. As it evaporates, your body feels cooler.

Bacteria makes sweat smell stinky! When the bacteria on your body mix with sweat, they start to grow and make it stink. When you take a bath or shower, you wash off the mixture of sweat and bacteria and then the smell disappears.

Protect Your Skin from the Sun

Sunburns hurt when you get them, and they can cause serious skin problems later in your life. You can protect your skin without having to stay out of the sun. Just remember these simple rules.

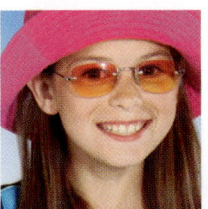

1. Wear a hat, shirt and sunglasses.

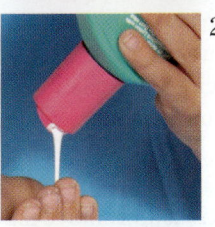

2. Put strong sunblock on skin that isn't covered. Use a sunblock year round. You can get sunburned in winter and on cloudy days.

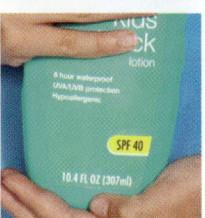

3. Make sure that the sunblock you use is SPF 15 or higher.

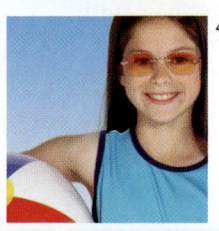

4. Use a waterproof sunblock if you play in water or sweat a lot.

Pimples and Zits

Some kids get pimples and zits when they approach their teens. Glands in their bodies produce oil that blocks pores and causes pimples and blackheads. If you have pimples on your face, wash your face gently and often – but don't scrub. You can't scrub the pimples away, and scrubbing makes them worse. Don't pick a pimple either.

If your pimples hurt or otherwise bother you, ask your parent to take you to your doctor who can help the pimples go away.

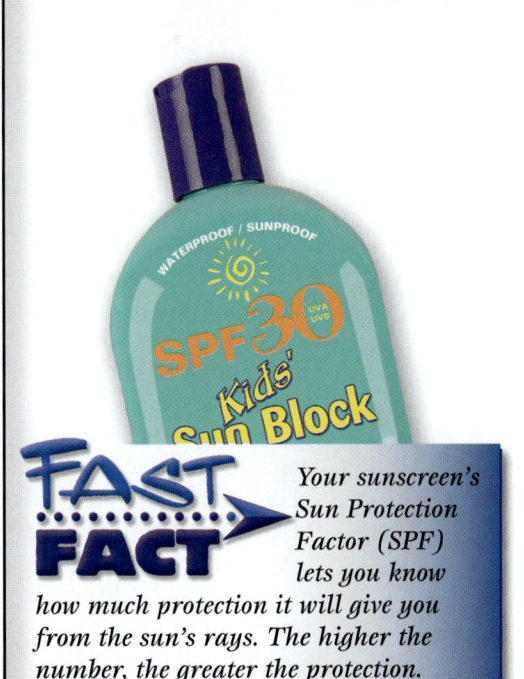

FAST FACT

Your sunscreen's Sun Protection Factor (SPF) lets you know how much protection it will give you from the sun's rays. The higher the number, the greater the protection.

Hair – Wavy, Curly and Straight

Redheads have around 80,000 hairs, brown- and black-haired people have about 100,000 and blondes have the most at 120,000! How should you take care of all that hair? Let's find out.

Keep It Clean
Some hair is oily, some is dry and some is just right. On average, kids wash their hair one to three times a week. If your hair seems oily or dry, tell your parent. You might need a special kind of shampoo or conditioner. If you have coarse or naturally curly hair, you might need special hair care products to help with tangles.

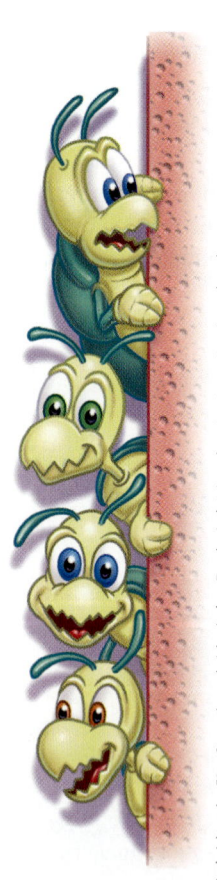

Critters
Most likely, you've heard about **head lice** – tiny insects that can live on your scalp and make it itch. Lots of kids get them, and it's nothing to be ashamed of. You can be the cleanest kid in the world and still get them. They can take a ride on a comb or jump from a hat that someone shares. You want to get rid of them right away because they lay eggs, called **nits**, which stick to your hair. The eggs make more head lice. Washing your hair isn't enough to kill them. You need a special comb to get rid of nits that attach to hair and a special shampoo to kill the lice. So, if you have an itchy head, or if you know that you've been around someone with head lice, tell a parent.

How to Wash Your Hair

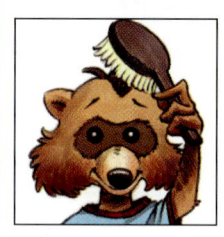

1. If you have long hair, brush it before you wash. This will remove tangles and surface dirt.

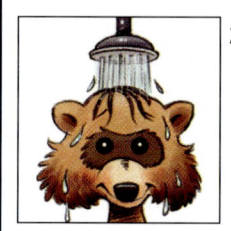

2. Next, get your hair good and wet.

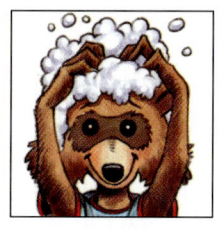

3. Lather it up with a mild shampoo or soap, and gently rub your head with the tips of your fingers.

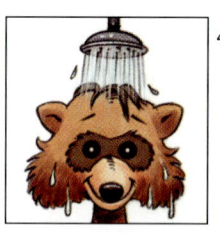

4. Rinse to remove all the suds. Leaving them there can give your hair a soapy build up.

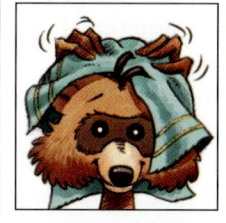

5. Dry hair with towel.

Sneezes, Sniffles and Coughs

Question: Which illness do you probably have most often, yet it has no cure?

Answer: The common cold! Many different viruses cause colds, but there are no vaccines or medicines to prevent or cure them.

The Truth About Colds
Most colds are caused by viruses called **rhinoviruses.** (The "rhino" part of the word comes from a Greek word that means "nose.") They can cause infections that affect your nose, throat, eyes and/or ears. Some can give you a slight fever and make you feel tired and cranky. You might have a sore throat, a sneezy and runny nose and/or watery eyes. You could also cough and feel chilly. Most of the time, your cold will end with a stuffy nose.

Rhinoviruses like to stay awhile. You'll probably feel sick within two or three days after the virus gets inside you and starts to grow. You are most likely to pass the cold to others during the first three or four days that you feel sick. Most colds last from one to two weeks. But the average is from five to seven days.

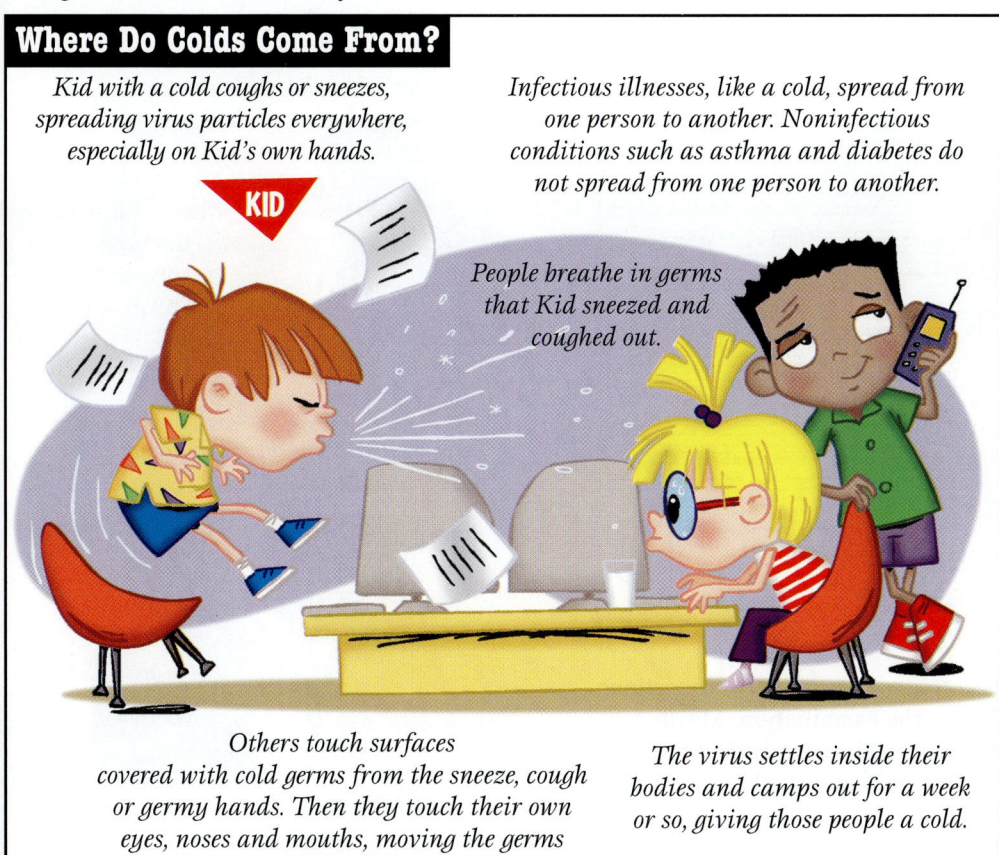

Where Do Colds Come From?

Kid with a cold coughs or sneezes, spreading virus particles everywhere, especially on Kid's own hands.

Infectious illnesses, like a cold, spread from one person to another. Noninfectious conditions such as asthma and diabetes do not spread from one person to another.

People breathe in germs that Kid sneezed and coughed out.

Others touch surfaces covered with cold germs from the sneeze, cough or germy hands. Then they touch their own eyes, noses and mouths, moving the germs inside their own bodies! Remember to always wash your hands.

The virus settles inside their bodies and camps out for a week or so, giving those people a cold.

The Doctor Is In

Even if you don't have a cold or other illness, you should visit the doctor every year for a checkup. Why? Because the doctor will make sure that all of your parts are healthy and strong, that you are growing correctly and that you know how to stay healthy.

What to Expect

At the doctor's office, your height and weight may be measured. You might be asked to get undressed, and the doctor may look and gently touch parts of your body. That's okay, the doctor just wants to make sure everything is okay.

The doctor will write things down in a special folder with your name on it called a **chart**. All the information about your health is in your chart.

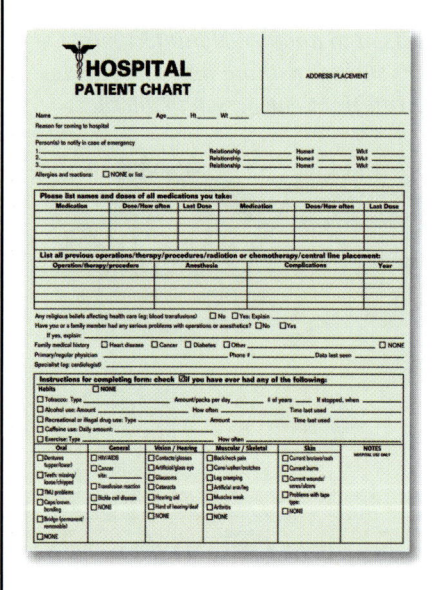

Feel free to ask the doctor questions during the examination. Maybe a part of your body hurts, or you are having problems at school or at home. Your doctor is your friend. He or she will tell you how to stay healthy, so pay close attention.

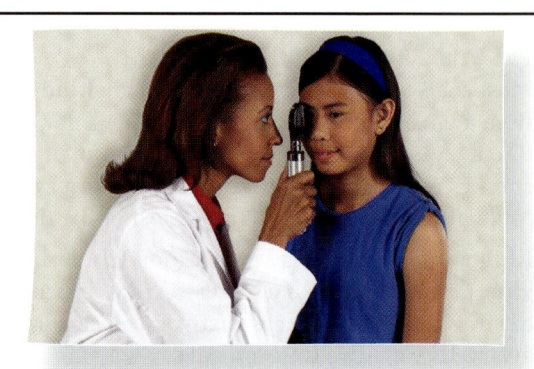

- **Eyesight and Hearing.** *The doctor wants to be sure you can see the board in school and hear what the teacher says.*

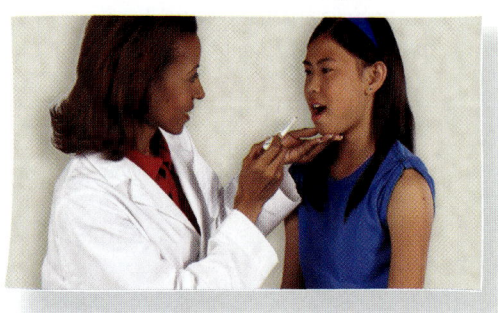

- **Temperature.** *The doctor may make sure that you don't have a fever.*

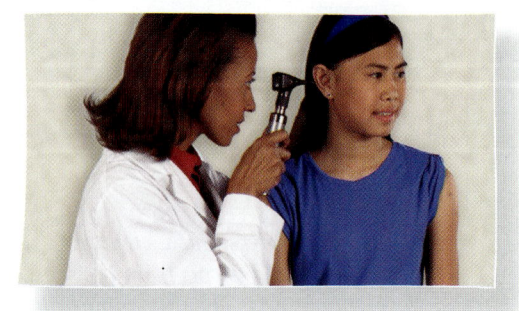

- **Eyes, Ears, Nose and Throat.** *The doctor will shine a light inside your ears, eyes and mouth to see what's going on in there.*

Pediatrician. What's That?

A **pediatrician** (pee-dee-a-trish-an) is a doctor who is specially trained to care for kids. In fact, you might see the same pediatrician all the way from babyhood to the age of 21. She or he will keep track of your growth and help you learn to become a strong, healthy adult.

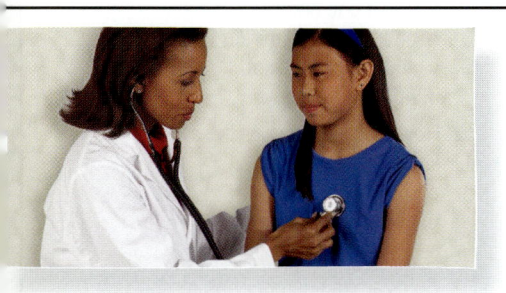

• **Heart and Lungs.** *The doctor will listen to your heartbeat and lungs while you breathe.*

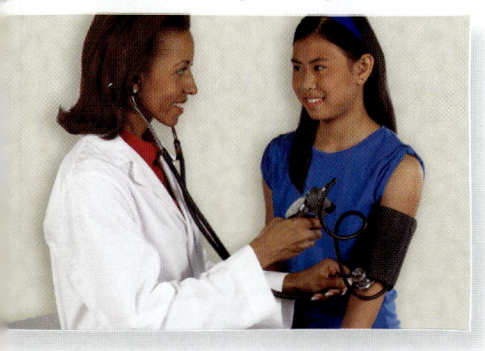

• **Blood Pressure.** *Your blood pressure will be checked to see how hard your heart is working.*

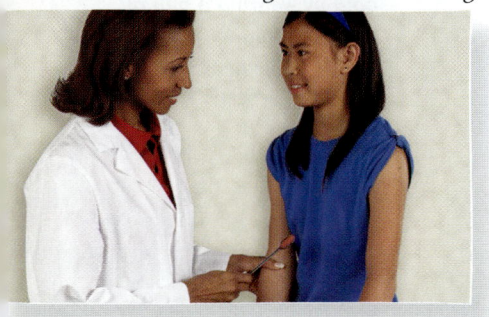

• **Muscles and Bones.** *Your doctor will tap your arms and legs with a little rubber hammer to test your reflexes. The doctor will also check your spine – the long, narrow bone that goes up your back – to make sure that it's growing straight and strong.*

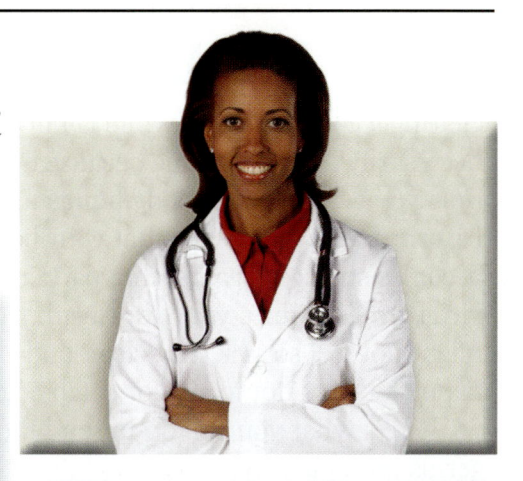

The Truth About Vaccines

You might need a shot to keep you from getting some serious germs that could make you very ill.

A shot is called a **vaccination** (vak-sin-ay-shun). It contains a tiny bit of the germ that could make you sick. The germ is fixed so it will not hurt you and your body can fight it off. When it does that, your body is protected from that germ. If you got a shot for chickenpox and then were around someone who has chickenpox, the vaccination would keep you from getting sick.

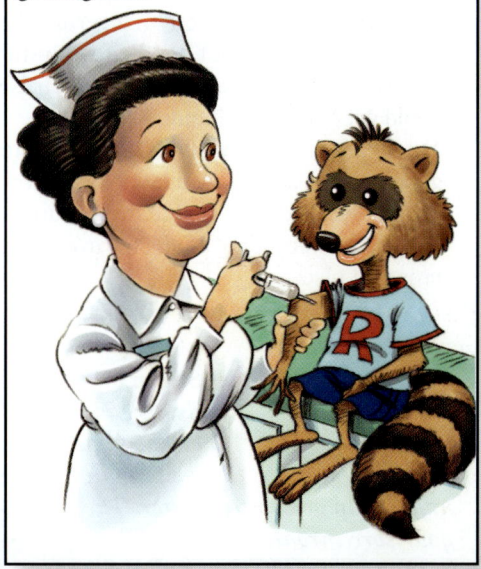

Oh, No You Don't!

Getting a cold once in a while is not necessarily an awful thing because every time you get one, your body builds up **immunity**. That means that your body becomes stronger against that particular virus, so if it comes your way again, you might not feel so sick. But clean and happy kids try not to give or catch colds. So, here's what you can do to send those germs on their way!

1. Wash your hands. Most colds are spread by germs left on surfaces when a person with a cold touches something. If you have a cold, or if you're around someone who has one, wash your hands often.
2. Use a tissue to cover your mouth and nose whenever you cough or sneeze. Then get rid of the tissue right away. Why? Because viruses can live for several hours on surfaces. If a thing covered with germs touches anything else, those germs will spread.
3. If you're caught without a tissue, cough or sneeze into the inside of your elbow. That part of you is least likely to touch something.
4. Get into the habit of not touching your eyes, nose or mouth when your hands aren't clean. Those are common places that germs like to enter your body. Don't handle food until you have washed your hands. The cold viruses could get from your hands to the food.
5. Eat healthy, drink plenty of liquids, exercise, get enough rest and try to stay away from people who are sick. If you are sick and coughing or sneezing a lot, stay away from crowded places.

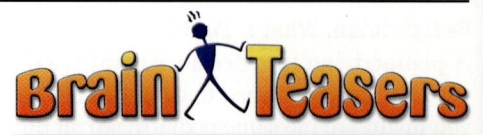

Brain Teasers

Colds

1. As a group, Americans get how many colds a year?
   a. about one billion
   b. about one-half million
   c. about fifty thousand
   d. none of the above
2. How many colds does the average kid get a year?
   a. six to eight
   b. one a month
   c. only three
3. Colds are the number one reason kids miss days at school.
   a. true
   b. false
4. A sneeze can_____.
   a. travel 100 miles per hour
   b. travel a distance of about 3 feet
   c. float in the air over 30 feet
   d. all of the above

Answers: 1. a; 2. a; 3. a; 4. d

If you were a kid in days gone by, you might have tried to cure your cold by wearing a bag of cooked onions around your neck.

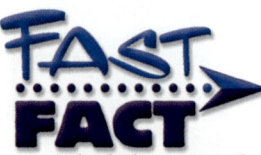

FAST FACT

Steam or salt water drops can unstuff your clogged nose. Chicken soup and other hot liquids might help you to feel better. They can soothe your sore throat.

Series Index

Pages are coded by book titles:
C - Clean Kids, Happy Kids
F - Fit Kids, Strong Kids
H - Hungry Kids, Healthy Kids
S - Safe Kids, Smart Kids

A
acid, C11
activity pyramid, C20-21
aerobic, F14, F18
alveoli, F17
arteries, F17
atria, F17

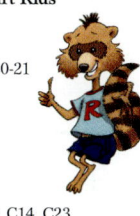

B
bacteria, C7, C11-12, C14, C23
bees, hornets & wasps, S18
biceps, F12
bike safety, S8-9
blood pressure, C27
blood vessels, C10, F17
bone marrow, F8
bones, C27, F8-12
booster seat, S7
breads & grains, H10-13
bronchi, F17
bronchioles, F17
brushing & flossing, C12-13, C16
bus safety, S7

C
calcium, C15, C17, F11, H18
calories, H28
camping safety, S16-17
cancellous, F8
capillaries, F17
carbohydrates, H7, H12
carbon dioxide, F16-17
cardiac muscle, F13
cartilage, F9
cavity, C11-12, C16-17
cementum, C10, C15
chambers, F17
chart, C26, C30-32, F30-32, H30-31, S30-32
checkup, C26
cholesterol, H28
cilia, F18
circulation, F16
clothing, F20-21
colds, C25, C28
cool down, F23
cortical, F8
crown, C10
cruciferous, H16
cusps, C10
cyber-strangers, S23

D
dental hygienist, C16-17
dentin, C10, C15
dentist, C16-17
digestion, H8
doctor, C26

E
electric current, S25
emergency (911), S28
enamel, C10, C15
endurance, F18
esophagus, H8
exercise, C20-21, F10, F15, F18, F22-F27

F
family fun, C21, F25
fats, oils & sweets, H7, H10-11, H22-23
fiber, H7, H13-14
fingernails, C9
fire safety, S26-27
fireworks, S27
fitness, C20, F6, F26-27, F30-31
fluoride, C11, C16
food groups, C14-15, C18, F10, F26-27, H10-11
food guide pyramid, C18-19, H10-11, H24-27
food labels, C15, H28
fruit, H10-11, H14-15
fungi, C7

G
germs, C7-9, C18, C25, C27-28
glucose, H12
glycogen, H12
gums, C10, C12, C17

H
hand signals, S9
hand washing, C8-9
healthy eating, C14-15, C18-19, F10, F19, F26-27, H24-27, H30-32
heart, C27, F13, F16-19
hemoglobin, H20
homogenizing, H19

I
ice & snow safety, S20
immunity, C28, C32
indigestion, H9
infections, C7, C25
iron, H20

J
jaw, C10
joints, F8-9, F14

K
kitchen safety, S24-25

L
lean, H20
ligaments, F9, F12
lungs, C27, F16-18

M
meat group, H10-11, H20-21
milk, yogurt & cheese, H10-11, H18-19
mosquitoes and ticks, S17
mucus, H7
muscles, C27, F12-15

N
neighborhood safety, S22
nerves, C10
nutrients, C15, H10

O
omega-3s, H20
orthodontist, C17
oxygen, F14, F16-17

P
pasteurizing, H19
peanut butter, H20-21
pediatrician, C27
plaque, C11

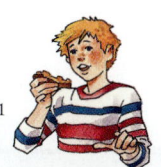

playground rules S12
poison ivy, S16
poison, S25
pores, C23
portion control, F19, H11, H19, H22
proteins, H7, H18
protozoa, C7
pulp, C10
pyrotechnician, S27

R
rhinoviruses, C25
root, C10

S
safe spots, S22
safety gear, F25
saliva, H8
saturated fatty acids, H22
scooter, skate & skateboard safety, S10-11
seatbelt, S7
serving size, C19, H11
showers & baths, C22-23
skeletal muscles, F13
skeleton, F8, F10-11
skin, C22
sledding safety, S21
smoking, F18
smooth muscles, F13
snowballs, S21
soap, C22
sodium, H28
sportsmanship, F28
starches, H13
stop, drop & roll, S26
storm safety, S15
street crossing, S8
stretching, F15, F22-23
sugar, C11, C14-15, H13, H23
sun protection factor (SPF), C23, F20-21
sunscreen, C23, F20-21
sweat, C23, F20
swimming safety, S19

T
teeth, C10-17
tendons, F9, F12
thunder and lightning, S14-15
tissue, C10
toenails, C9
trachea, F17
triceps, F12

U
unsaturated fatty acids, H22

V
vaccination, C27
vegetables, H10-11, H16-17
ventricles, F17
villi, H9
virus, C7, C25, C28
vitamins & minerals, F8, H7, H14-17, H20

W
warm up, F22
water, H7

X
X-rays, C17

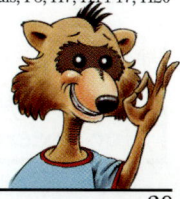

29

Take the Clean Kids Challenge

For the next week, work on completing the chart on these pages. Each day, check off the healthy habits you've practiced and write the number of times you did them. You will do some things each day. Others you might only do when needed.

Healthy Habits	Sunday	Monday	Tuesday
Washed My Hands			
Brushed My Teeth			
Flossed My Teeth			
Cleaned My Nails			
Ate Healthy Foods			
Got Some Exercise			
Took a Bath or a Shower			
Washed my Hair			
Covered my Mouth or Nose When I Coughed or Sneezed			

If you forget how often you should do each of these things, review the information in this book.

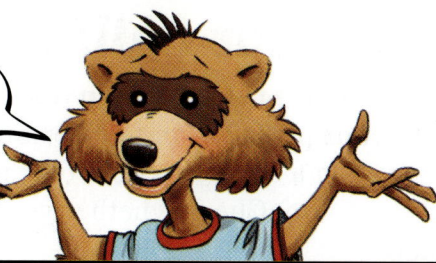

Wednesday	Thursday	Friday	Saturday

Parents: Your Child's Immunizations

Use the handy chart below to keep track of your child's immunizations. Check with your pediatrician to determine your child's specific needs, which depend on a child's age and overall health. Adults and teens need immunizations also. Check whether you are up-to-date when you visit your doctor.

Types of Immunization	Dates	Name of Provider	Other Information
Hepatitis B			
Diphtheria Tetanus, Pertussis (DTP)			
Tetanus and Diphtheria			
Haemophilus Influenzae type b			
Poliovirus			
Measles, Mumps, Rubella			
Chickenpox (Varicella)			
Pneumococcal Disease (PCV)			
Hepatitis A			
Influenza			
Meningococcal			